An Insider's View of
Bipolar Disease

An Insider's View of

BIPOLAR DISEASE

HOW TO RECOGNIZE THE SYMPTOMS, UNDERSTAND THE TREATMENTS AND SOLVE THE CHALLENGES TO LIFE, RELATIONSHIPS AND CAREER

PAUL GOLDEN, M.D.
THE BIPOLAR PHYSICIAN

Dudley Court Press
Sonoita, AZ

Published in the United States of America by:

Dudley Court Press
P.O. Box 102

Sonoita, Arizona, 85637 USA
www.DudleyCourtPress.com

Paperback ISBN: 9781940013183

Kindle ISBN: 9781940013190

"I think you're brave to ask for help."

Author's daughter, to her father

Contents

INTRODUCTION *11*

QUESTION 1
What is bipolar disease? 13

QUESTION 2
What is depression? 17

QUESTION 3
What is mania? 21

QUESTION 4
What is the depression side like? What does it feel like? 23

QUESTION 5
What is the manic side like? What does it feel like? 25

QUESTION 6
What is the difference between major depression and the blues?
..... 29

QUESTION 7
How do you know if you are manic and not just overly enthusiastic?
..... 33

QUESTION 8
What are Personality Disorders? 35

QUESTION 9
What is the difference between bipolar disease and schizophrenia?
..... 39

QUESTION 10
Are you responsible for someone with bipolar disease? What should
you do? 41

QUESTION 11
What treatments are available? 45

QUESTION 12
What is ECT and is it still used? 51

QUESTION 13

   *Are there alternative treatments? **57***

QUESTION 14

   *How do you find the right treatment? **59***

QUESTION 15

   *How does stress affect people with bipolar disease? **63***

QUESTION 16

   *Is bipolar disease hereditary? **67***

QUESTION 17

   *Is there a higher risk of suicide? **71***

QUESTION 18

   *What famous people have had major depression or bipolar disease?
   ..... **73***

QUESTION 19

   *How do you manage a career if you have bipolar disease? **77***

QUESTION 20

   *How do you deal with the social stigma? **83***

CONCLUSION **91**

ABOUT THE AUTHOR **93**

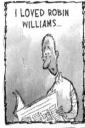

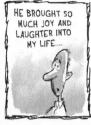

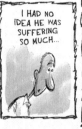

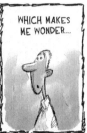

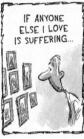

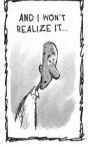

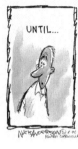

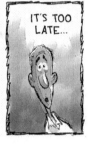

Introduction

For hundreds of years, anyone with mental illness has been stigmatized. It's time for society in the twenty-first century to learn the subtleties of the term "mental illness" and stop the stigmatizing. I used to think it was my parent's and earlier generations that preserved the negativity. Now, I find that my peers, even my medical colleagues, still harbor misunderstandings and negative prejudice towards people with mental illness. Through this book I want to change that.

I am going to focus on "affective disorders," also called mood disorders. These consist of bipolar disease and unipolar major depression. The myriad of other mental disorders will be brought into the discussion to differentiate them from affective disorders. Having bipolar disease for over forty years, I am most comfortable with this area.

People with bipolar disease can become successful working members of society at all levels. This book is not about me. It is about those of us who have conquered this albatross of mental illness with medicines and talk therapy. I want to give hope to those whose lives have been turned upside down.

Part of my mission is to highlight the need for broader access to care for those affected by mental illness. Restriction of access to psychiatrists and psychologists by insurance companies, Medicare and Medicaid is a serious problem

People with mental illnesses such as bipolar disease, major depression and co-existing anxiety disorders fall into a very large crack in our society and do not have access to psychiatric care, proper education about their disease, or a spouse/friend as a support partner. Also, to be frank, many people with these conditions do not try to seek help. However, proper care, education and a support system are needed for societal success, just as in the treatment of diabetes or congestive heart failure and other chronic conditions.

I do not announce to the world that I have bipolar disease. However, over the years my peers, doctors, friends, family and some patients have learned of my mental disease. They know the quality of my work and accept me for who I am. I know that life with bipolar disease can be satisfying and productive and I want to encourage you to believe your life can be satisfying and productive too.

Often people with bipolar disease are highly intelligent, amazingly functional and live high profile lives. I will highlight Winston Churchill, Mahatmas Gandhi, Abraham Lincoln, Ernest Hemingway, Virginia Woolf and others who suffered from bipolar disease.

If you or someone you love suffers from bipolar disease, I encourage you to start here to learn more about the disease. Learn what treatments are available. Learn what it feels like to experience the ups and downs of bipolar disease. And learn how to live a full and productive life despite the challenges of living with bipolar disease.

Reach out to me at www.mdgolden.com if I can be of further help. You are not alone.

Paul Golden, M.D.
The Bipolar Physician

Question 1

What is bipolar disease?

~

Bipolar disease is a mood disorder and was previously referred to as manic-depressive disease. According to the American Psychiatric Association's Diagnostic and Statistical Manual, the two major mood disorders are **unipolar major depression** and **bipolar disease**.

There are two categories of bipolar disease, bipolar I and bipolar II. The difference is a matter of the severity of the manic component. Bipolar I is the more severe form, with major depression and mania. Bipolar II involves major depression and hypomania — 'hypo' means less severe. In bipolar I, destructive symptoms and borderline psychotic features are present. *(Solomon, D.A., et al, Archives of General Psychology, 2010; 67:339-347* Many with bipolar disease have coexisting anxiety or other "personality disorders" that will be discussed later. *(Merkarios, K.R., et al, AGP, 2007; 64)*

Bipolar disease involves both depressive and manic states. Manic behavior includes rapid thoughts, which can be positive or negative, fast speaking, feeling superior than others, being the life of the party with quick improvised joking, increased desire for sex, buying sprees, etc. The most destructive component is irritability, which can lead to fights and borderline psychotic behavior if left untreated. *(Jamison, K. and Goodwin, Manic-Depressive Disorder, 1990, pages 4-6)*

The cause of bipolar disease and major depression is unknown. We do know that an imbalance of serotonin, dopamine and norepinephrine, all neurotransmitters, exists in the brain when bipolar disease and major depression disease are present. Treating these imbalances is the basis of the therapies.

It is not clear if childhood factors of abuse or family history of suicide may contribute to the existence or severity of the disease.

Rapid cycling, i.e., episodes of depression and mania that occur weekly or even daily, reflects a severe form of bipolar disease. "With rapid cycling, mood swings can quickly go from low to high and back again, and occur over periods of a few days and sometimes even hours. The person feels like he or she is on a roller coaster, with moods and energy change that are out of control and disabling. In some individuals, rapid cycling is characterized by severe irritability, anger, impulsivity, and uncontrollable outbursts." *(Bipolar Disorder: Rapid Cycling and its Treatment, Depression and Bipolar Support Alliance (DBSA), 730 N. Franklin Street, Suite 501, Chicago, Illinois 60610-7224, phone 800-826-3632)*

According to this same report, it is rare for the first episode of bipolar disease to present as rapid cycling. Also, about one-half of bipolar patients will have an episode of rapid cycling during the course of their disease. A link with substance or alcohol abuse is suggested.

Rarely, features of mania and depression occur at the same time; this is referred to as a 'mixed state.' This subgroup is the hardest to treat but fortunately the least common.

The usual age of onset of major depression or bipolar disease is in the third decade. However over the past ten to fifteen years, both are occurring at earlier ages. Often a patient experiences major depression and is treated only for that. With the powerful drugs now available for major depression, sometimes the treatment triggers a manic state, which then leads to a diagnosis of bipolar disease.

Question 2

What is depression?

~

Depression is a state of feeling sad or despondent or down in the dumps. The intensity or seriousness of the state of depression determines whether it is just a case of the blues, mild chronic depression, situational depression or major depression. It's not always easy to determine precisely what kind of depression a patient is experiencing. In fact, one study indicates that most patients see their primary care physician first and the diagnosis, at least of major depression, is missed. *(Mojtabal, R., et al, J. of Clin Psych 2009; 69:1064-1074*

Major depression is the most serious form of depression and requires treatment from a knowledgeable medical professional.

Major depression is defined as having at least five specific symptoms that last at least two weeks. The possible symptoms which can combine to indicate major depression include: feelings of sadness, emptiness, pessimism, feeling guilty and worthless, agitation, hopelessness, early day awakening, obsessing, not wanting to get out of bed, gain or loss of weight, suicidal thoughts, lack of interest in hobbies, difficulty functioning and making decisions, fatigue, and inability to concentrate. *(Judd, et al, JAMA, Psychiatry 2013; 70:1171)*

The usual age of onset of major depression is in the twenties but a more precise median is thirty-two years of age. Each year 6.7% of U.S. adults experience an episode of major depression. Women experience major depression twice as often as men. More than 3% of adolescents 13 to 18 years of age have had a life-disrupting episode of major depression and this number is rising.

Major depression can be divided into four subtypes:

1. Major depression
2. Persistent depressive disorder—major depression or less severe symptoms for two years
3. Psychotic depression—major depression plus psychotic symptoms (delusions)
4. Postpartum depression—10 to 15% of women
5. Seasonal affective disorder—major depression worse in winter months and improved in spring and summer months when natural sunlight abounds. UV light therapy can help in the winter but often patients will be on medications during the dark time of the year. *(The National Institute of Mental Health: www. nimh.nih.gov/health/topics/depression/index. shtml)*

Generally, major depression is not the result of external life events such as loss of a family member. It is endogenous, meaning coming from within and occurring for no reason, out of the blue, per se. The community standard for treatment of major depression includes three modalities: talk therapy with a psychologist, psychiatric care and medications. This is the case in bipolar patients as well. *(Kessler et al: Development of life-time co-morbidity in the world WHO mental health surveys. Arch. Of Psychiatry 2011; pages 68-100.)*

Question 3

What is mania?

Mania and hypomania are not stand-alone diseases. Mania is half of what defines bipolar disease. The other half is major depression disease. Hypomania is a milder form of the manic episode. Some people in a manic phase do not want the good feeling to stop and therefore do not take their medications. They are highly productive when manic, but there is a very dark side to mania — irritability. The latter can get people into a lot of trouble.

A manic episode is a period of elevated mood lasting more than two weeks and perceived as abnormal for that individual. Friends can observe it before the patient. Patients' goals change from hour to hour or even less. Impairment of judgment in the work place, home or school eventually leads to lack of the ability to function.

Unlike in major depression, a manic episode is not caused or exacerbated by substance abuse such as illicit or legal drugs, alcohol or a life event. Three or more of the following symptoms must coexist:

1. Rapid speech
2. Racing thoughts
3. Aggressive behavior
4. Irritability

5. Risky behavior

6. Spending sprees

7. Poor financial choices

8. Drive to complete multiple projects

(http://www.mayoclinic.org/diseases-conditions/ bipolar-disorder/basics/symptoms/con-20027544)

There is no such thing as just being manic or hypomanic alone. The closest to such a personality would be hyperthymia. As described in his blog, David Joel Miller describes such individuals as people who have so much energy and get so much accomplished that they may become annoying to others. "Hyperthymia has been defined as equivalent to hypomania but without the impairment." *http://counselorrssoapbox.com/2012/06/07/ hyperthymia-hyperthymic-personality-disorder-and-bo- lar-disorder/*

Question 4

What is the depression side like? What does it feel like?

~

While everyone has their own way of describing their experience of major depression, there are many similarities in what happens. When I experienced major depression for the first time, I felt buried alive. I dreaded each day. My self-confidence was shot. I lost my appetite. I felt like someone sucker-punched me in the stomach, again and again. I could barely get out of bed each morning.

Others comment that the experience of major depression is "like someone with an army boot is pressing down on my chest;" "like trying to run up a hill of mud and always sliding down;" "movement and thinking are in slow motion;" "I can't make decisions;" "I have crying jags;" "I cannot smile;" "I cannot concentrate." *www.// ncbi.nlm.nih.gov/pmc/articles/PMC486942/*

The author William Styron describes his personal experience during his first major depressive episode in the book, *Darkness Visible*. He writes: "It was not really alarming at first, since the change was subtle, but I did notice my surroundings took on a different tone at certain times: the shadows of nightfall seemed more somber, my mornings were less buoyant, walks in the woods became less zestful, and there was a moment during my working hours in the late afternoon when a kind of panic and anxiety overtook me…"

The poet Edna St. Vincent Millay writes in "Burial" of being "six feet deep." In "Sorrow," she likens sorrow to "ceaseless rain …People twist and scream in pain in a chair." And she declares, "The anguish of the world is on my tongue. My bowl is filled to the brim with it."

Mike Wallace of *60 Minutes* fame wrote in his book, *On the Edge of Darkness*, "People who don't know [what depression is] who say it's self-indulgence, sound callous, but it's not callousness born of indifference; I think it's callousness born of ignorance. That kind of ignorance we've got to get rid of, and little by little I suppose, we will. You say to them, 'It's a pity you don't know. I'm sure that if you knew, I'M SURE THAT IF YOU KNEW, not only wouldn't you say that, you'd try to help in one way or another."

Question 5

What is the manic side like?
What does it feel like?

~

The individual experience of mania varies, of course. The pattern, however, is predictable. Mania begins with super-positive energy that eventually turns to irritability with others and the world which, fueled by the same over-the-top intensity, can lead to destructive behavior. It can take years to realize and anticipate the pattern.

A good understanding of this can be seen through the eyes of Juliet, as described on the website, Healthy-Place.com. Regarding hypomania she writes, "I feel joy juice surging through my veins.... A colossal 'high' has found me. I'm witty, charming, quick, talkative and effervescent.... Euphoria is an understatement. I want to share this feeling with everyone so I compulsively call people randomly on the phone while chatting on the computer.... I'm chatting with strangers, shopping for things I don't need."

When she is in a manic stage, she experiences what many do — sleeplessness, or rather a lack of interest in sleeping because action and thinking take over. "I haven't been to sleep in three days. I'm buzzing down the road erratically and much too fast behind the wheel of a car I have no business driving. ...My irritability is off the

Richter scale. My mind is racing, things are jumbled, and I am not making clear conversation."

When you are in a manic phase, you are amazingly productive, new ideas come fast. In her book, *Manic-Depressive Illness*, Dr. Kay R. Jamison puts it this way: "The ideas and feelings are fast and frequent like shooting stars and you follow them until you find better and brighter ones. Shyness goes, the right words and gestures are suddenly there, the power to seduce and captivate others a felt certainty.... Sensuality is pervasive.... Feelings of ease, intensity, power wellbeing, financial omnipotence and euphoria now pervade one's marrow. The fast ideas are too fast and there are far too many.... Humor and absorption on friends' faces are replaced by fear and concern.... You are irritable, angry, frightened ... Madness carves its own reality." In that last sentence she is saying that left untreated, mania can result in auditory or visual delusions, i.e. psychosis.

An indication that something is wrong is the strong desire to keep the euphoria going. The consequences of the euphoria are trivialized or denied as in this first person narrative: "The mania part is awesome. I have tons of energy and don't want to stop. The best part of mania is that I'm so optimistic about everything.... Getting into a fistfight at a bar with some dude twice my size is exhilarating. I know it's destructive, but it's the greatest form of entertainment because it's raw, tough and totally dangerous. I've yet to be seriously hurt in one of these fights, so I keep escalating each time. It's like a game to me." *(Healthline, January 4, 2012. "In Their Shoes: Understanding What Bipolar Disorder Feels Like")*

Question 6

What is the difference between major depression and the blues?

~

According to The National Institute of Mental Health the difference between major depression and the blues can be described this way: "Everyone occasionally feels blue or sad. But these feelings are usually short-lived and pass within a couple days. When you have major depression, it interferes with daily life and causes pain for both you and those who care about you. Major depression is a common but serious illness." *(www.nimh.nih.gov/health/ publications/depression/index.shtml)*

Major depression episodes can occur with no apparent reason. The despair associated even with getting out of bed in the morning is overwhelming. The feelings of hopelessness, of no way out, of nothing but bleakness…these are the hallmarks of major depression.

Contrast the intensity of such despair and bleakness with, say, the feeling of disappointment or feeling 'bummed out' when you get a C on a term paper when you were expecting an A.

Other terms for everyday "depression" or blues are **situational depression** or **exogenous depression.** Exogenous means 'coming from without.' Situational or exogenous depression is a response to a negative circumstance or life experience, i.e., a rainy day at your wedding or that lousy grade.

Endogenous depression, on the other hand, is a synonym for major depression, and "means coming from within." It happens for no external reason.

It's likely that every one of us has experienced, at one time or another, some form of depression ourselves, or someone near to us has. Nurses, doctors, police, fire fighters, military personnel, prison workers, wardens, deputy sheriffs, lawyers, judges, and volunteers at homeless shelters and with the Salvation Army, United Way, or Goodwill often come face to face with both major depression and situational depression in the people they serve, but may not know the difference. Only major depression is a mental disease!

Priests, ministers, rabbis and clerics advise members of their churches, temples and mosques who suffer from major depression and situational depression but they, in particular, need to know the difference between major depression and grief.

Anyone suffering major depression deserves appropriate treatment. However, it is my contention that today, too many people are being treated with drugs for situational depression just like too many people are being treated with antibiotics for conditions for which they are not appropriate.

Take the following analogy: A patient comes into the office or calls with the following symptoms: yellow nasal discharge, fatigue, cough, no fever. Likely this is just a cold or viral bronchitis and treatment is fluids, rest and over the counter cold medications. Juxtapose this with a patient with productive cough of green phlegm, fever of 101 or higher, headache and body aches. They need antibiotics because the infection is bacterial.

When patients who don't need them are given antibiotics, they may suffer unnecessary side effects and, worse, resistant bacteria become a risk for society overall. All too often, however, patients want pills and doctors oblige.

Similarly with mental conditions, too often patients want pills, and doctors oblige. Determining the kind of depression a patient is suffering from too often falls to primary care physicians today. Distinguishing between situational depression, major depression, bipolar disease or even schizophrenia can be very challenging. Family practitioners and internists are pressed by the big pharmaceutical industry's television commercials to prescribe drugs. Patients see the same commercials and follow the commercial's instructions to "Ask your doctor for XYZ drug." These drugs have potential serious side effects so are not to be thrown around lightly, particularly when the diagnosis is unclear.

Most patients who 'feel depressed' are suffering from prolonged grief (perhaps from the loss of a family member) or from a severe health problem or simply feel 'down' for a week or so due to circumstances in their life. These issues are not going to respond to drug therapy unless the individual already has a history of bipolar disease or major depression or this prolonged episode is actually a first-time episode of major depression.

The distinction between situational depression and major depression can be blurry. Either the patient should be referred to a psychologist for talk therapy or, if the physician digs deeper, he or she may find that a patient with situational depression has a family history that includes schizophrenia, institutionalization, seasonal symptoms where the blues are worse in winter and gone in summer, or a distant family member who has committed suicide. It can be helpful, in these cases, to try drug treatment. However, if the individual does not see a difference in six weeks, he or she should be taken off the medicine because it is not helping and could have deleterious effects.

The moral imperative is to be sure of the diagnosis.

Question 7

How do you know if you are manic and not just overly enthusiastic?

For individuals who suffer with mania, the onset of the first manic or hypomanic episode is very difficult to recognize. Sometimes even after multiple episodes, it's hard to understand the seriousness of the problem. Often a spouse or good friend is the first to alert you that you are making the transition into the clinical status of mania.

Only in retrospect did I realize that from about 1966 I was crossing the line between too enthusiastic to manic. There were times when my fast thinking, fast doing and fast joking were not normal, although I thought I was just energetic. The first of my three major depressive episodes occurred in 1973 but mania wasn't actually diagnosed until 1987.

Synonyms for enthusiastic include words like energetic, forceful, kinetic, aggressive, gung-ho, lusty, mettlesome, impetuous, charged up, vitriolic, and animated. Any of those synonyms for enthusiastic could apply to people who are manic.

So you can see the conundrum. How is the average layman able to tell the difference? How can I tell the difference? How can anybody with bipolar disease tell the difference?

"This is the challenge, then, and the defining aspect to mania — being unable to recognize when you have crossed the line from exhilaration or irritation to being out-of-control. If you keep escalating the exhilaration/irritation, you will hurt yourself, disrespect yourself, or hurt others emotionally or physically. Suddenly your spouse sees thousands of dollars on a credit card, or worse. A newly manic individual is likely to go on to societal acts of mayhem and greater explosivity. This leads to more risk of suicide, more hospitalizations and poorer prognosis." *(Bellani, M. et al, J.Psych.Research 2012; 46:616-621)*

When the enthusiasm becomes problematic in terms of personal relationships and ability to function in normal society, one should consider the possibility of a diagnosis of mania.

If you've never been diagnosed with bipolar disease but you have experienced episodes of depression, and now someone tells you that your behavior seems 'manic', or that you are speaking too fast, or you are too energetic, or you feel your thoughts are coming too fast, you should consider the possibility that you are actually bipolar. You should talk with your doctor.

If you know you have bipolar disease, and a family member or good friend tells you that you are starting to 'fly high', they are probably correct. You need to learn not to get angry or defensive. Instead, seek professional help.

Question 8

What are Personality Disorders?

Many people wonder if depression or bipolar disease are considered to be personality disorders. They are not. Although they are all forms of mental illness, depression and bipolar disease belong to a group of disorders called mood, or affective disorders. Personality disorders are another group or class of mental illness. Sometimes people have more than one mental illness so someone who is depressed might also have a personality disorder. This is similar to someone having more than one physical illness. For example, someone with an endocrine disease like diabetes might also have a respiratory disease like emphysema.

I recall reading the book *Girl Interrupted* by Susanna Kaysen. The book came out in 1993. It is autobiographical and set in 1967 when she was admitted to a private institution in Massachusetts. She had taken an overdose of sleeping pills.

As I first read the book I was confused about what her actual diagnosis was. Years later, after practicing medicine a few years, I understood what 'personality disorder' meant. Susanna Kaysen's personality disorder, Borderline Personality Disorder, was characterized by impulsivity, difficulty with interpersonal relationships and self-image, fears of abandonment, anger and irritability. Self-harm is particularly characteristic of this personality disorder.

The other personality disorders are:

- Schizoid Personality Disorder — introverted, withdrawn, emotionally cold and distant
- Paranoid Personality Disorder — perceiving actions of others as threatening and therefore untrusting.
- Schizotypal Personality Disorder — need for social isolation, anxiety in social situations, odd behavior and thinking, and often unconventional beliefs.

- Anti-social Personality Disorder — ignore normal rules of social behavior, irresponsible and callous, legal issues and irresponsible behavior.

- Narcissistic Personality Disorder — increased sense of self-importance, unlimited success, seek constant attention, oversensitive to failure, has multiple somatic (physical) symptoms and exploit what few people they call friends.

- Avoidant Personality Disorder— hypersensitive to rejection, need reassurance of being liked, and may have no close relationships outside their family circle

- Dependent Personality Disorder — pattern of dependent and submissive behavior relying on others to make decision for them.

- Obsessive-Compulsive Personality Disorder — marked by high levels of aspiration, very conscientious, strive for perfection, orderly, methodical, inflexible to adapt to any change in routine, cautious, detail oriented and have difficulty completing tasks.

- Histrionic Personality Disorder — need attention, needs to be the center of attention, dramatic, acting out a role to others that makes keeping close sexual relationships difficult, crave novelty and bored with routine and use physical appearance to garner attention. *(www.mentalhealthamerica.net/ conditions/personality-disorder)*

It's important to diagnosis the specific personality disorder because each has a slightly different treatment protocol. Psychologists are usually the first line professionals to treat personality disorders.

Question 9

What is the difference between bipolar disease and schizophrenia?

~

Schizophrenia is a mental illness that is different from other mental illnesses. Schizophrenia is set apart from all other mental disorders by *psychosis*. Psychosis means auditory, visual or olfactory (smell) hallucinations. In addition it is the most crippling of all mental diseases as it leads to social withdrawal and impaired functioning, particularly in the educational and workplace environments. Accordingly, it is one of the most crippling of all diseases. *(Murray, C.J., et al, The Global Burden of Disease, Harvard U. Press, Cambridge, Mass. 1996 pg. 21).*

Abnormal speech cognition, flat affect, paucity of speech, memory and higher cognitive function make up just part of the disease. Delusions other than of the senses, but at times involving the senses, could be everything from being Jesus to being an alien. Auditory delusions could be in the form of a voice directing a task. *(The Diagnosis and understanding of schizophrenia. Parts I, II and III, respectively by Carpenter, Batko and Strauss, Schizophrenia Bull, 1974: 37, 50 and 61)*

Delusions can also be described as paranoid, grandiose and erotic, all three of which are likely to lead to major legal/criminal issues. Catatonia, although usually thought of as stillness, can also be repetitive behavior to frank muteness. Delusions without any intent is known as simple schizophrenia.

Onset can be sudden or gradual; symptoms, continuous or remitting; long-term, poor versus non-poor prognosis. Surprising to me is that most patients in one study had an acute onset, intermittent symptoms and only mild symptoms in the long run. *(Modestin, J. et al, Long term course...Am J. Psychiatry 2003:160:2202-2208)*

More relevant to the subject of mood disorders is the association of depression with schizophrenia. As I have noted elsewhere, people with a mood disorder often suffer with another mental illness as well. Approximately 25% of patients with schizophrenia also have major depression. *(Conus, P. et al, Pre-morbid correlates of first episode mania or depression with psychosis...J. Affect Disord 2010; 126:88-95)*. Risk factors for the coexisting disorders are mostly hereditary. Depression in this setting can be depression (melancholia type), unipolar depression or Major Depression disease. (Amer. Psych. Assoc. 4th text revision, Washington, D.C.)

Treatment with anti-depressants does not conclusively change outcome in schizophrenia. *(Siris, S.G. et al, Arch of Gen Psych 1987; 44:533-539)*, (Whitehead, C., et al, Antidepressants for people with both ... Cochran Data Base of Systematic Reviews, 2002; CD002305). Typically, the traditional antipsychotics such as Haldol, Thorazine and Navane or the atypical (new) antipsychotics such as Zyprexa and Abilify are the standard of care.

Question 10

Are you responsible for someone with bipolar disease? What should you do?

~

First you must recognize that bipolar disease is a treatable illness caused by chemical imbalances in the body, not unlike diabetes. Diabetes affects the pancreas. Bipolar disease affects the brain. The disease is real and you can't expect someone to 'snap out of it.' However it is serious and potentially life-threatening, and needs to be treated with professional care.

The signs of untreated bipolar disease have been described in the previous Questions 1-7.

If you are responsible for someone with the disease, you can find support at the Depressions and Bipolar Support Alliance (800-826-3632). They point out that "you can't make your loved one well, but you can offer support, understanding and hope."

They suggest the following steps:

1. Educate yourself

2. Give unconditional love and support.

3. Encourage him or her to get professional help.

4. Be patient, and take care of yourself too

5. Offer to go along for appointments

If you think the person might be considering suicide, call 911 or call a Hotline 800-442-HOPE and remove all weapons from the home.

Sometimes, when symptoms of depression or mania become severe, it's necessary for a person to be hospitalized. The emergency room of the closest hospital may do a preliminary evaluation and then refer the patient to a psychiatric hospital. If the patient is deemed a danger to themselves or others, they may be required to stay in the hospital for a seventy-two hour hold.

I'm writing this book just after the unfortunate suicide of comedian Robin Williams. From the first time I saw him perform, in the movie "Good Morning Vietnam" I was sure he was bipolar. His improvised humor and fast repartee, which we all saw during many of his appearances on talk shows, were clearly manic in my opinion.

For all his known problems with cocaine and alcohol, there was never any mention of depression or of his seeing a psychiatrist or taking psych medicines. The only medications in his system that were found through an autopsy were one for sleep and one for Parkinson's.

His friends knew he was hurting, particularly as his talent waned in movies and in the world of television. He had to sell a large piece of property in Marin County where he grew up and lived. He also had been told he had early Parkinson's. Yet no mention of his fight with depression was made until after his death.

Was this another tragedy of a brilliant artist with bipolar disease whose friends and family either didn't recognize or refused to deal with the symptoms? Like so many other artists with bipolar disease, his genius was wasted. He was only sixty-three years old. I would love to read a biography of this amazingly talented man someday. And I hope that someday the family will come forward with what was really going on behind the scenes as far as psychiatric issues. It would do society a great service.

Who is responsible for this tragedy — the man, the disease or his loved ones?

One of the big challenges is to get a person with bipolar disease to act.

I went to my haircutter recently. She proceeded to spend the whole hour not only cutting my hair but talking about her husband's doctor, his meds, and his diagnosis. Her husband was being treated for bipolar disease. I've known Mary a long time. I had treated her father and mother in my nephrology practice and Mary knew I was bipolar and would likely know the answers to her questions.

Mary's husband was on lithium, Abilify, Geodon, Cymbalta and recently Adderall. She said he was tremulous, had no facial expression or desire to do anything. I asked her if he walked without swinging his arms. (This is a side effect of antipsychotic medicines such as Abilify or Geodon.)

She nodded yes. I went over an inventory of symptoms of Major Depression, Bipolar Disease and Schizophrenia. It became obvious Mary's husband had Major

Depression only. If he were bipolar, the Cymbalta would make him worse and the two atypical psychotics were the cause for his zombie look and his persistent hand movements, as well as his Parkinson's like walk.

Indeed, he had all the side effects of the old antipsychotics Haldol and Thorazine. We used to have a saying in residency that anyone who could tolerate Thorazine was indeed schizophrenic.

What Mary started out asking me was how she could get her husband to see a different doctor. I gave her two names and said if she could not convince him, then she should call me.

At the end of the haircut I gave Mary the usual twenty-five dollars and said maybe she should pay me. That gave us both a good laugh. Unfortunately, I learned during my next haircut that Mary's husband refused to see a different doctor.

It can be frustrating to be close to someone with bipolar disease who doesn't listen to advice that could help them improve their functioning. The best you can do is try.

Again, if a person's situation is very serious and you think the person might be considering suicide, call 911 or call a Hotline 800-442-HOPE and remove all weapons from the home.

Question 11

What treatments are available?

Lithium is the primary drug used in the treatment of bipolar disease, although new drugs are made available all the time. Lithium is the first in a class of drugs known as mood stabilizers. Mood stabilizers lengthen the interval between episodes of mania and depression, and maintain the patient in a normal (euthymic) state. Lithium is better at reducing manic attacks but also downgrades serious depression episodes as well.

Lithium has an interesting history. In the 19th century, it was discovered that water from certain mineral springs in Texas, when ingested, caused improvement in manic patients. These "crazy waters" contained high levels of lithium carbonate. *(Fowler, G. Crazy Water: The Story of Mineral Wells and Other Texas Health Resorts. Fort Worth: Texas Christian University Press:1991)*

In 1847 a British physician, Alfred Garrod, discovered that uric acid was present in excess in patients with gout or gout kidney stones. To dilute the urine, Garrod used lithium. *(Garrod, AB. The Nature and Treatment of Gout and Rheumatic Gout. London: Walton:1859).*

The modern use of lithium to treat mania can be pinpointed to 1949 when John Cade, reviewing Garrod's work, felt that uric acid had a connection to mania and started using lithium carbonate and lithium citrate on manic patients. He had remarkable success, with some patients being able to be discharged from institutions after years of unsuccessful treatment. *(Cade, J., et al, Lithium salts in the treatment of psychotic excitement. Med J Aust. 1949; 2:349-352).*

Many case reports of success in many countries led to the use of lithium carbonate for the mania aspect of bipolar disease. By 1954 studies showed equal efficacy to ECT with the mere prophylactic use of a pill. The administration was tricky until blood levels could be measured, which was achieved in 1958. *(National Institutes of Health. Office of NIH history. Laboratory instructions Collection. Museum of Medical Research, October 2006).*

Lithium's use in the U.S. was slow to take on but by the late 1960's, as blood levels could be easily measured, it became the treatment of choice for prevention and treatment of the manic side of bipolar disease as a 'mood stabilizer.'

Lithium's side-effects include tremor, uncommon cardiac arrhythmia, thyroid dysfunction and renal insufficiency. The importance of frequent blood level checks cannot be overstated as the difference between a therapeutic versus toxic level is very small. *(Canada, final publication PubMedCentral, Bipolar disorder Jun 2009; 11 Supp. 2:4-9)*

The mechanism of action in Lithium remains elusive. It seems to affect various parts of the central nervous system neurons. An enzyme inhibited by lithium is involved restoring the body's clock known as circadian rhythm and Lithium can also raise serotonin levels. *(Rao,*

JS et al; Mol. Psychiatry 13 (6)585-596). Now it has been shown that Lithium prevents swings in both directions, manic and depressive.

～

The first medications used for the treatment of depression were Tricyclics, thus named because their molecules are made of three components. The Tricyclics first came into use in the late 1950's and were the only drugs until the SNRIs (selective norepinephrine reuptake inhibitors such as Wellbutrin) came out in the late 1980's. Selective serotonin reuptake inhibitors (SSRIs) became popular in the early 1990's.

Zoloft, Prozac, Lexapro, Paxil and others are among these breakthrough medications introduced in the '90s. The mechanism of action of SSRIs acts right at the core cause of major depression. Depression is caused by an excess of serotonin in the brain. The SSRIs block this buildup of serotonin.

The combination SNRI/SSRI drugs Effexor, Cymbalta and Pristiq block both neurotransmitters. These are the ideal drugs for major depressions patients. However, not all patients respond the same way to medication so trial and error becomes the ART of medicine. *(Mclroy, SL et al, Yatham, L.N., et al, Bipolar disorder: 2013:15:1-44)*

A major caveat in the treatment of bipolar disease is not to use SSRIs or the combination drugs alone. They are too potent and will likely flip a major depression episode to mania in bipolar patients. It is recommended that monotherapy be avoided in bipo-

lar disease. *(Pacchiarotti I, et al, Amer. J. Psychiatry 2013:170:1249-1262)*

~

Anti-seizure drugs such as Tegretol were a therapy for bipolar depression in the past. Newer anti-seizure drugs Depakote and Lamictal are now at the forefront to treat bipolar disease but as add-ons or in lieu of therapy with lithium for bipolar disease. *(Viktorin, A. et al, Am J.of Psychiatry:171:10:Oct 2014).*

The new atypical antipsychotics, Zyprexa, Seroquel, Abilify and Geodon were originally for use only for schizophrenia. They are now used with lithium for bipolar disease and as add-on therapy for major depression if the SSRIs are not bringing patients back to their normal feeling. These have replaced the traditional anti-psychotics, Haldol and Thorazine. The side effects of all of the antipsychotics are significant but occur to a lesser degree with the newer drugs.

The side effects of antipsychotics include a pseudo-Parkinson state and an "antsy" feeling. Side effects also include repeated muscle movements, such as lip smacking, over which the patient has no control. Sometimes even when the drug is stopped, the side-effect can persist.

One last thing about every antidepressant from Tricyclics to SSRIs/SNRIs is they all have the potential to cause suicidal ideation and suicide and should not be used in adolescents.

The consensus is that combination therapy with lithium, low dose antidepressants, atypical antipsychotics, and new seizure medicines, talk therapy (psychologists) and ECT (discussed in Question 12) make up the armamentarium for the treatment of bipolar disease. *(American Psychiatric Association: Practice Guideline for the treatment of Major depression alone and/or bipolar disease, Third Edition, 2012:4, 17 (NIH & Clinical Excellence:90:2010.)* A recent approach in the treatment of bipolar disease is to use Lithium or Limictal as single drug therapy as there is some anti-depressant and certainly anti-manic features to them.

Some experimental modalities are undergoing clinical trials. These include ketamine, deep brain stimulation and ablative neurosurgery. *(Keller, M.B. et al, J of Clin Psychiatry 2005:66 Supplement 8:5-12).* They are definitely radical and most of us would just tell patients that they have a chronic disease that cannot be cured, but can be managed. This means taking your medications, exercising regularly, maintaining healthy sleep habits and coping.

A concern for treatment of children and teens is a bit up in the air. Generally the same meds are used but the numbers of cases treated this way may not have been carried out long enough to know if other side-effects will occur. Psychotherapy and teaching coping skills certainly would be first-line approach. Most do not use SSRIs as there is a chance for actually increasing suicidal ideation and suicide itself.

Question 12

What is ECT and is it still used?

ECT or electro-convulsive therapy is very much a major therapeutic tool in the treatment of stubborn major depression. ECT is the passage of a small amount of electricity from one temple through to the other with two small paddles. Unfortunately, the method is still very much vilified by the public.

Ken Kesey's "One Flew over the Cuckoo's nest," published in 1962, gives a negative spin to ECT. The main character McCarthy has himself deliberately transferred from the prison system to the psychiatric system by feigning mental problems. His behavior is so outrageous that he earns himself ECT treatments. A swaggerer and gambler, he continues to bait Nurse Ratched to the point that he is forced to have a frontal lobotomy and at the end is quiet, almost drooling, and mute and without feeling. Kesey experienced some of this first hand in an Oregon mental hospital in 1952.

The evolution of ECT as practiced today went through several earlier and unpleasant origins.

"The History of Shock Therapy in Psychiatry" by Renato M.E. Sabbatini, PhD *(http://www.cerebromente. org.br/n04/historia/shock-i.htm)* goes into depth, specifically, on insulin shock therapy. Between 1917 and 1935 there were actually several ways to insult the central nervous system into inducing seizures.

It was observed that head trauma, seizures and fever improved symptoms of mental patients in the insane asylums of the past, specifically manic and schizophrenic patients who had been incarcerated for long periods of time. Dramatic return to normalcy allowed for the release of many patients.

In and around 1917 Dr. Wagner-Jauregg found that "insane" patients improved after developing infections from typhoid fever. The most common malady in asylums were patients suffering from the third stage of syphilis, neuro-syphilis, which includes mania, paralysis, dementia, motor coordination, speech deficits and ultimately death. Malaria-induce fever seemed to improve the neurological symptoms of syphilis. The connection between the malaria parasite and a type of mosquito in 1895 allowed for creating fever in the syphilitic patients.

Insulin given to induce coma and seizures was first used to treat schizophrenia in Berlin by Manfred J. Sakel in 1927. Insulin itself and its role in modulating glucose (sugar) levels had only just been discovered in 1921 by two Canadians. Sakel accidentally found that by inducing coma and seizures with an overdose of insulin (insulin shock therapy or ICT), symptoms of psychosis improved greatly. Called "Sakel's Technique" it became the routine for treating schizophrenics in Vienna in 1930 and then in the U.S. in 1934. In a 1939 study of 1700 cases of schizophrenia, there was complete or partial improvement in sixty-three per-cent using this treatment. *(M.J.*

Sakel (1956) The classical Sakel shock treatment: a reappraisal. In F. Maarti-Ibanex et al. (eds.) The great physiodynamic therapies in psychiatry: an historical reappraisal. New York: 13-75)

Meanwhile in 1933, a Hungarian named Ladislau von Meduna tried various chemicals injected intravenously and found a hydrogen and nitrogen-based molecule metrazol to create convulsions. The convulsions were too severe, causing multiple fractures despite minor changes in dosing. *(C Allen, 1949:* Modern discoveries in medical psychology. *London: 219-20)*

Finally, in 1937 ECT was used for the first time by Drs. Cerletti and Bini in Rome. They were convinced that seizures work but the inherent danger of insulin and Metrazol led them to create seizures by passing electricity across the head. Stigma still exists because of the early methods which did not employ general anesthesia or muscle relaxers.

After trial and error, Cerlettin and Bini settled on a methodology and frequency of treatments. They found that ten treatments on alternate days was optimal. The only side-effect was loss of memory for a short period after the shock (called retrograde amnesia) which was beneficial as there was no pre-procedure anxiety. Bini and Cerletti's machine was introduced around the world and became widespread in use during the 1950's. Researchers were actually more impressed with its effectiveness on mood disorder patients. *(Shorter, Eward (2007). A History of Electroconvulsive Treatment in Mental Illness. New Brunswick, N.J.: Rutgers University Press. Pp. 46-47).*

ECT has been shown to have a 65% remission rate compared to the use of medications. *Surgeon General (1999). Mental Health: A Report of the Surgeon General chapter 4. and from Prudic J, Olfson M, Marcus SC, Fuller RB, Sackeim HA (2004) "Effectiveness of electorconvulsive therapy in community settings". Biol. Psychiatry 2004: 55 (3): 301-12.*

ECT is also considered one of the least harmful treatments for severely depressed pregnant women because of the potential deleterious effects of medications on the pregnancy and the fetus. *(Miller L.J. (May 1994) "Use of electroconvulsive therapy during pregnancy" Hosp Community Psychiatry 45 (5):444-450*

ECT replaced insulin and Metrazol as the treatment of choice for affective disorders and schizophrenia. Gradually refinements with muscle relaxers and short-acting sedatives, oxygen, and seizure monitoring with a brain wave machine (EEG) led to the procedure we know today. Between 150,000 and 200,000 procedures a year are performed in the U.S.

Some famous people who have received ECT include Dick Cavett (TV host), Paulo Coelho (author), Thomas Eagleton (U.S. Senator), Carrie Fisher (actress), Ernest Hemingway (author), Vladamir Horowitz (pianist), Vivian Leigh (actress), Yves St. Laurent (designer).

Negative reaction to ECT was due to its overuse with resistant or troublesome patients who were shocked several times a day, often without restraints or sedation.

In addition the most refractory Bipolar or Major depression patients (the ones that do not respond to pharmaceuticals), tend to be the older age group and they respond best to ECT. There is no specific number of treatments but the consensus is between six and twelve on Mondays, Wednesdays, and Fridays. *(Amer Psych Assoc Task Force on ECT: Washington D.C. 2001)*

Question 13

Are there alternative treatments?

Patients have asked me about "holistic," or "alternative treatments" for bipolar disease. Although I'm not an expert in this area, I think there are many options for reducing stress and mood triggers in one's life. By combining professional medical treatment for bipolar disease with alternative or complementary treatments, you may reduce the intensity of depressive episodes or the onset of them. I do meditation with my white toy poodle every day outside on a bench out at the round-about in our community. It gives me quiet time and 'time-outs' which I have found help me immensely.

Remember that bipolar disease is a chronic condition with no known cure. However there are definitely things you can do to ease the symptoms and reduce the impact of triggers that can induce depressive or manic cycles. You can add these alternative treatments and lifestyle changes but DO NOT RELY ON ALTERNATIVE TREATMENTS ONLY. Bipolar disease is a biochemical condition that needs professional treatment.

Besides meditation, other lifestyle changes you can make to reduce the intensity of depression and stabilize your moods include:

- moderate exercise,
- identifying and reducing stress in your daily life,
- avoiding over-the-counter drugs that can contribute to depression (e.g., antihistamines and others),
- avoiding recreational drugs, including alcohol and illegal substances,
- reducing intake of caffeine and sugar, both of which contribute to mood swings.

You can also consider adding supplements like B vitamins or St. John's Wort and be sure to eat a nutritious, well-balanced diet.

Relaxation therapy, biofeedback, massage therapy, acupuncture, yoga and even light therapy can offer help to someone with bipolar disease. In northern latitudes such as Alaska or Norway, the long winters can cause routine depression or melancholia as well as major depression. In a patient with unipolar major depression or bipolar disease the effect is orders of magnitude greater, as is the risk for suicide.

Full spectrum lights are useful for folks with or without mental diseases who live in climates with long, dark winters, or who spend most of their days indoors. Available as headlamps or desktop lamps, these full spectrum lights help with mood disorders when used daily for about 30 minutes.

Question 14

How do you find the right treatment?

Medications now are the primary treatment for bipolar disease and of major depression. However, I have to take a stand here. I believe that the power of the pharmaceutical companies and media to influence the excessive consumption of drugs — not just for depression but for erectile dysfunction, diabetes, insomnia and even complicated acting drugs for rheumatoid arthritis — represents capitalism at its worse. The new drugs coming out almost daily make it confusing to patients who are inundated by commercials on television.

The problem with psychiatric drugs is the major overlap and duplication among them. All these drugs fall into the same four classes of agents and add nothing of value to most of us — except to the pockets of pharmaceutical companies.

Primary care providers, usually an internist or family practitioner, are the first line of treatment for people struggling with any mental illness. Unfortunately, the medical insurance system often blocks access to psychologists and psychiatrists who are trained to deal with mental illnesses in ways that primary care providers are not. This is a big problem. Primary care providers vary tremendously in their training and ability to handle these complex diseases, let alone to know which medications to use.

If you or your loved one has already experienced depression or is being treated for depression, ask these questions to illuminate the possibility of bipolar disease:

- Have you ever had episodes when other people think you are talking too much, too fast, or changing subjects too quickly?
- Have you ever had episodes of spending too much money quickly?
- Have you engaged in risky sexual behavior?
- Have you made risky investment choices?
- Have you had episodes of speeding in your car without concern for safety?
- Have you had episode of being too energetic or productive, to the point of being irritable with other people?

Although some of these behaviors may be defined as hypomanic, left untreated in someone who experiences depression, they can become full blown manic episodes, which can be ruinous to your life and loved ones. Recognizing these signs of bipolar disease early and getting proper treatment is critical.

For mild to moderate unipolar depression and for bipolar disease or major depression, psychotherapy should be the first line of treatment. Psychotherapy involves one-on-one guidance by a psychologist or psychiatrist to help a patient eliminate unhealthy habits, negative beliefs and negative behaviors. Family therapy and group therapy are also goal-directed and use a psychologist as moderator.

Likewise, relaxation therapy including breathing exercises are good adjunctive therapy.

As far as prescription drugs go, lithium and its history have already been discussed in great detail. Lithium became a worldwide treatment for bipolar disease in 1949. In addition to asking the questions listed above to confirm a diagnosis of bipolar disease, your doctor should measure certain blood levels before prescribing lithium. Such tests as renal (kidney) function, urinalysis, a pregnancy test for women of child-bearing age, EKG and thyroid function are essential. *(Am J Psychiatry. Apr 2002;159(Supp 4)1-50).* These tests should be repeated periodically.

If lithium alone does not reduce the manic symptoms, the next approach could be to add Lamictal, one of the newer anti-seizure agents, to an antidepressant such as Prozac or Zoloft, in small doses. As a rule of thumb, changing one drug at a time is optimal.

For patients who just do not respond to any medications, ECT is largely effective, as described in Question 12.

The CDC (Center for Disease Control) publishes information about mental health, the burdens of mental illness, and mental health basics at http://www.cdc.gov.

Question 15

How does stress affect people with bipolar disease?

~

Stress is a word that is often misunderstood today. Stress is pressure, tension or strain. Stress can affect people with bipolar disease just as it affects everyone. We all live with mental stressors throughout our lives. The issue is how one deals with stress. Getting into a car accident, fear of flying and getting a bad grade can all create stress but none of these lead to major depression or bipolar disease.

Dr. Nassir Ghaemi, in his book *A First- Rate Madness-Uncovering the Links Between Leadership and Mental Illness* (Penguin Books 2011) noted a study of the well-being of 2000 adults. He reported that, despite experiencing at least one of thirty-seven harmful life events such as losing a loved one, most people do not suffer much depression "even with severe stress." (pg. 127) As physical stress builds muscle, or vaccines create resistance to diseases, emotional stress can build greater capability to weather difficult situations in the future. Ghaemi offers a metaphor: "Trauma itself is not a disease, just as a virus is not itself an infection." (pg. 128)

In bipolar depression stress causes muscle tension, reduced immunity, epinephrine surge and emotional stress that can reduce ability to weather difficult situations . Stress does not cause bipolar disease but can exacerbate it.

If you become anxious due to a stressful situation, then you experience anxiety. Anxiety is a sensation, and emotional reaction, that comes from within. It is a fact that bipolar disease often coexists with an anxiety disorder. Stress can exacerbate anxiety.

At a conference of the Anxiety and Depression Association of America, Naomi Simon, M.D., Associate Director of Anxiety and Traumatic Stress Disorders at Massachusetts General Hospital said that making a diagnosis of an anxiety disorder, bipolar disease, or both together can be tricky. She stated some clues involve: panic attacks with severe anxiety coexisting with bipolar symptoms, childhood onset of anxiety disorder with subsequent development of Bipolar disease, problems with sleep and anxiety even when not in a depressed or manic state and, surprisingly, patients who have more difficulty finding a medical regimen that works. Bipolar disease with anxiety disorder is a double hit leading to decreased quality of life, likeliness of substance abuse and suicide. Severe insomnia (of itself an anxiety disorder) can trigger manic attacks.

A discussion of bipolar disease in geriatrics has a bit of a different spin to it but if you read between the lines the role of anxiety versus stress is no different. The prevalence of bipolar disease in adults over sixty-five in the U.S. is one in one hundred in one year. *(Kessler, R.C. et al, Arch of Genl Psychiatry 2005;62(6):593-602)* Older patients with bipolar disease had many more stressful life events. Remember, the word is STRESSFUL, but this is the geriatric population.

It is clear that bipolar disease in the geriatric population is different from younger patients. Co-existing anxiety is more common. *(Sajatovic, M. et al, Geriatric bipolar disorder. Psych. Clin. North Am 2011; 34:319-333)* Also co-existing diseases such as diabetes, hypertension, heart disease, chronic lung disease are hugely more common in the geriatric population.

Anxiety disorders (not stressors) occur in ten percent of patients with geriatric bipolar disease such as agoraphobia, anxiety disorder, panic attacks and others. *(Sajatovic, M. et al, J. of Geriatric Psych 2006; 21:582-587)*

Question 16

Is bipolar disease hereditary?

~

Dr. N Ghaemi, previously referenced in question 15, states that bipolar disease is the most hereditary of the mental disorders, being more so than schizophrenia and major depression. If you have a parent or sibling with bipolar disorder, there is a 15% chance that you will develop it. If you have a second-degree relative like an aunt or grandparent, then the incidence is about 7-8%.

Mendlewicz, J. and Rainer *(Br J Psych 1972; 120:523-530)* showed that offspring of one bipolar parent have a median of 10% chance of developing the disease. If both parents have the disease, their children have a 30% chance of developing bipolar disease. This is in comparison with 0 to 2% of children of parents who do not have the disease.

It's important to note that if a first or second-degree relative with bipolar disease has been treated successfully with a particular drug regimen, a patient is more likely to respond to the same drug regimen. *(Gartiehner, G. et al, Curr Psych Rep 2012; 14:360)*

On the other hand, other studies show that there are more than one gene abnormality accounting for not only the hereditary tendency but also the observation that the inheritance is lower than expected. *(Crad-*

dock, N., et al, Genetics of bipolar disorder. Lancet 2013; 381:1654-1662)

In 2010, the National Institutes of Health (NIH) reported that researchers found a gene "hot spot" for both bipolar disorder and major depression. McMahon et al, combined studies to analyze 13,600 people and confirmed that Chromosome 3 variations were associated with both mood disorders.

Newer data from the NIH has now shown that five major mental illnesses can be traced to a group of genetic variations. Studies reflecting work at 80 research centers in 20 countries reported overlap of gene variation in all five illnesses. The strongest correlation came from studies of twins.

Studies of family history, identical twins, fraternal twins, and twins separated at birth by adoption showed inherited tendencies at play with a highest incidence of bipolar disease in identical twins raised in different homes. *(Neuberger, Jul., Jr. et al, Arch. Gen Psych 2011; 68:1012-1020).*

If one identical twin is bipolar, the chances are high (55-70%) that the other twin will also be bipolar. This incidence is consistent whether the twins are raised together or separately, in their biological home or an adoptive home.

In an incredible look back on same sex twins from 1870 to 1920 in the Danish Twin Registry, Bertelsen and colleagues in 1979 reported that identical twins born between 1870 and 1920 had a sixty-seven percent incidence of manic-depressive illness compared to twenty percent for fraternal twins of same sex. *(Bertelsen A., London: Academic Press, 1979:227-239 and Br J of Psych 1977 130:330-351)*

On a more positive note with respect to family planning, children with one bipolar parent have rates of 4% to 15% of developing bipolar disease compared to 0% to 2% when neither parent has the disease. If both parents are bipolar, a child has a 3.5 times greater chance of being bipolar than if only one parent is bipolar. (www.health.com/health/condition-article/0,,20275258,00.html)

Question 17

Is there a higher risk
of suicide?

Yes, unfortunately. Approximately 15 to 17 percent of people with bipolar disease will commit suicide, compared to about 1% of the general population and approximately half of all bipolar patients will make at least one suicide attempt in their lifetimes.

People with bipolar disorder who are not treated, or who are not treated properly for the disease are at a much higher risk for suicide than people who do receive treatment.

Suicide usually occurs during the major depression phase of the illness. According to the Treatment Advocacy Center (www.treatmentadvocacycenter.org), "The extreme depression and psychoses that can result from lack of treatment are the usual culprits..."

It's important for you to realize that the 85% of bipolar patients DO NOT commit suicide. The most important preventive measure is good treatment. If you or someone you love shows the symptoms of bipolar disease or major depression, get treatment as soon as possible.

Here are some resources specifically related to suicide prevention:

Suicide Chat Hotline, Chat anonymously 24 Hours/Day, www.remedy live.com/

24 Hour Crises Hotline, www.emqff.org/services/crisis

National Suicide Prevention Lifeline, www.suicidepreventionlifeline.orag/

Need help? In the U.S. call 1-800-273-8255

California Youth Crisis Line, www.youthcrisisline.org/

Question 18

What famous people have had major depression or bipolar disease?

～

People with bipolar disease and major depression can take some solace in the highly intelligent, creative artists, leaders, philosophers, writers and politicians who have been or have been diagnosed with either of the above diseases.

There is evidence that these diseases go back to the Greek playwright, Aeschylus who, born in 525 B.C., is known as the Father of Tragedy. In his plays, he is equivocal about whether major depression is hereditary or not. His plays represent dark, gothic tales of major depression. It is from his most famous play, *Agamemnon*, that the quote "He who learns must suffer. And even in our sleep, pain that cannot forget falls drop by drop upon the heart, and in our own despair, against our will, comes wisdom to us by the awful grace of God."

Read Kay Jamison's book *Manic-Depressive Illness and The Artistic Temperament* for an in-depth look at individuals down through time with bipolar disease or major depression. Also read her memoir, *An Unquiet Mind: A Memoir of Moods and Madness,* about her own battle with bipolar disease as she strived for her goal of a Ph.D.

in Psychology and eventual Professorship in Psychology at Johns Hopkins School of Medicine. Jamison also co-authored with Frederick K. Goodwin, M.D., a must-read treatise on the disease itself, *Manic-Depressive Illness: Bipolar Disease and Recurrent Depression* 2007 (2nd edition.)

A stunning and disquieting short memoir by William Styron (author of *Sophie's Choice*) is almost too uncomfortable to recommend to one experiencing their first major depression. However, his *Darkness Visible, A Memoir of Madness* could be valuable reading for someone dealing with someone they love who suffers from depression.

Notable others and their biographies include the following:

> Benjamin Franklin — *The First American: The Life and Times of Benjamin Franklin*, H.W. Brands. 2000
>
> Douglas MacArthur — *American Caesar*, William Manchester, 1978
>
> T.E. Lawrence — *Lawrence & the Arabian Adventure*, Robert Graves, 1928
>
> Virginia Woolf — *A Writers Diary, Extracts from the Diary of Virginia Woolf*, edited by Leonard Woolf (her husband) 1953.
>
> Virginia Woolf — *Virginia Woolf: The Impact of Childhood Sexual Abuse on Her Life and Work*, Louise DeSalvo, 1989

Rebecca West (the early twentieth century British author) — *A Life*, Victoria Glendinning. 1987

William R. Hearst — *Citizen Hearst* by W.A. Swanberg, 1961

Franklin Delano Roosevelt — *The Privileged Life of and Radical Presidency of Franklin D. Roosevelt*, by H.W. Brands, 2008

Edward Teller — *Teller's War; The Top Secret Story Behind the Star Wars Deception*, William j. Broad, 1992

Earnest Hemingway — *Hemingway*, Kenneth S. Lynn, 1987

Winston Churchill — *The Last Lion, Defender of the Throne*, William Manchester and Paul Reid, 2012

John Nash — *A Beautiful Mind: The Life of Mathematical Genius and Nobel Laureate John Nash*, Sylvia Nasir, 1998

Woodrow Wilson — *Dead Wake, The Last Crossing of the Lusitania*, Erik Larson, 2015.

How do you manage a career if you have bipolar disease?

The last two questions in this book are at the heart of my venturing into this project. The fact is, bipolar disease, along with all other mental illnesses, carries a stigma that can negatively — though often unjustifiably — impact your career. I address the issue of social stigma further in Question 20. For now, I'd like to address the career issue. I can give some gut feelings and some factual information.

First, I would say neither be transparent nor opaque, but rather translucent about volunteering information on your history with these diseases. What I mean is, don't be a victim of your own honesty; be strategic and be prepared. There are two arenas I want to address — your medical information and practical considerations for career choices.

Revealing Your Medical History

Regarding your medical information, if you are under the treatment of a primary care physician only, and either bipolar disease or major depression is suspected, you must find a way to be referred to a psychiatrist. Your relationship with your psychiatrist is critical to preserving your privacy, and preserving your privacy is essential to managing your career when you have bipolar disease or major depression or any other mental illness. Do not sign a HIPPA release that has your psychiatrist's name on it. Only sign a HIPPA release with your primary care physician's name.

Your primary care physician should know the name of your psychiatrist and should know about the psychiatric medications you are taking. However, your primary care physician does NOT need to know any details about your psychiatric history. You can tell him or her that you prefer to keep that information confidential between you and your psychiatrist. You have the right to instruct your primary care physician NOT to disclose the psychiatric history information. You might provide the information (your psychiatrist's name and the list of psychiatric medications) on a separate piece of paper with the statement: "Confidential. Not to be released under any circumstances."

Be careful when you see a new doctor of any specialty or are applying for disability or life insurance. You may be asked for a list of medications that you are taking or about prior hospitalizations, or the names of your doctors. Consider how forthcoming you want to be with information regarding psychiatric issues. I feel it's perfectly appropriate to leave out information about psychiatric medications. I don't think it's necessary to provide the name of your psychiatrist. I believe it's appropriate to give the name of one's primary physician only. I recommend that you don't volunteer information about hospitalizations relating to psychiatric care.

The only time it is important to release the names of your medications is when you are hospitalized for any reason because medications do impact your medical or surgical care. This, of course, removes the cloak of privacy. However, you can be pro-active by asking each person who interacts with you these two questions: "Do you feel comfortable caring for me?" and "Can you keep the information about my psychiatric history confidential?"

Career Practicalities

As for career practicalities, it's a good idea to know your limitations before settling on a career. If you're going into medicine, for example, pick a nine-to-five specialty such as dermatology or endocrinology, particularly if you have the primary obligation in your family unit as breadwinner. You need to be in a medical specialty that carries less stress and more flexibility so that you can more easily manage your life with bipolar disease.

In whichever career choice you make, you need to be able to respond to advice from family or your doctor, especially, "You need to take time off." Your career needs to allow for occasional time off on the advice of your psychiatrist or when your body says you need it.

Recognize that changes in time zones or challenges to your circadian rhythm make management of your condition more difficult. So carefully weigh these concerns as you consider a career that involves significant travel or night shifts or changes to your routine.

If your career requires a state or federal license, you need to understand what the application process requires and you need to be prepared to decide what you will or won't disclose. Applications vary from state to state and from license to license. Should you lie if asked to supply information on prior or present history of mental diseases? That is a personal decision, but realize you may eventually be caught in the lie so you need to know the consequences. (*A National Analysis of Medical Licensure Applications, Sarah J. Polfliet, M.D., Journal of the American Academy of Psychiatry and the Law, September 2008, vol. 36; number 3: 369-374*)

Study the American with Disabilities Act (ADA), which was signed into law in 1990 but is not strictly followed. Since 2006, most state licensing boards ask for mental health history. Some licensing agencies specify a time limit. For example, they ask "In the last five years have you ever been treated for a mental illness or taken medicine for one?" If you are applying for law enforcement or the military, the question is not if you have a mental illness, but rather have you ever been treated with a psychiatric medicine.

The American Psychiatric Association (APA) has a position paper stating that any such questions regarding physical or mental disabilities stigmatizes applicants. (*ADA position paper: Washington D.C. American Psychiatric Assoc. Dec 1997*)

Regarding the application, renewal or removing licensure of a physician, cases that have gone to the Circuit Court of Appeals using Title 2 of the ADA have regularly found in favor of the physician. But who has the money to go through the process? And who wants the public disclosure that comes with this process? *(New Jersey in 1993: Circuit Court of Appeals Using Title II of the ADA found in favor of the physician and Hason versus Medical Board of California, 1995)*

My conclusion is, if you are considering a career in any field that requires a license, be prepared for obstacles.

Under current U.S. disability law, it is not legal to fire someone already in medicine, law, nursing or teaching unless "problem behavior develops." If you are in those fields now, do your research to understand how "problem behavior" is defined in your area.

Be aware of laws regarding your psychiatrist's obligation to reveal to your employer that you are a "danger to yourself or others." Laws regarding patient confidentiality are changing and differ in each country and, in the U.S, from state to state.

It is a different world out there compared to my generation. Our children and grandchildren face far greater stress finding employment. Most have some albatross to carry through life. I feel that it is now more difficult for the millennial generation. Even the process of applying for blue-collar jobs can be fraught with stress, not only because of the application but also due to background checks and drug testing.

In her book, *Adult Bipolar Disorders*, Mitzi Waltz provides excellent advice on the following issues relating to employment: preparing for applications and interviews, enforcement of non-discrimination laws, the Federal Rehabilitation Act, medical leave, help getting a job, career choices, off-limit occupations, low stress work options and, finally, to "Out at work or Not." I recommend this book as intelligent self-defense and wise preparation.

The ultimate tragedy involving these disorders and career was the crash of the Germanwings commercial jet, a subsidiary of Lufthansa in early 2015. While debate continues about privacy versus disclosure rules, I want to speak directly to those of you who, like me, have bipolar disease, and the responsibility we have to step up to the challenge of living with this condition.

The co-pilot of the Germanwings jet was twenty-seven at the time of the crash. The major depression he suffered in 2009 when he was twenty-one years old might have been his first, which can be terrifying and seem like a life-ending experience. Although the co-pilot was forthcoming then, his fears for the career he dreamed since his teenage years may have subsequently led to years of subterfuge. His self-stigma, secrecy and concern for his career reflect a life lived without a social conscience. He didn't accept his disease and its limitations. He didn't learn how to regulate himself, nor did he have a support group to help him make the right decisions. His personal tragedy extended to become a horrific social tragedy.

Don't let your life go in that direction.

Question 20

How do you deal with the social stigma?

When you know you have to live with bipolar disease or major depression, you quickly realize that in addition to the diseases, you also have to live with the stigma they involve. Stigma is defined by the Oxford Dictionary as "a mark of disgrace associated with a particular circumstance, quality or person." Miriam Webster also defines stigma as a "set of negative and often unfair beliefs that a society or group of people have about something." It is these unfair, negative beliefs about bipolar disease and the people, like me and you who have it, that I want to challenge. By publishing this book, *An Insider's View of Bipolar Disease* and my memoir, *Functional Bipolar: 39 Years a Physician*, I wish to lessen the stigma attached to bipolar disease and major depression.

Stigma in the military

The NIH has studied stigma in active duty military personnel with bipolar disease or major depression compared to National Guard troops with those conditions three and 12 months after returning from combat in Iraq. *"Stigma barriers to care, and use of mental health services among active duty and National Guard soldiers after combat," Km Py, et al, Psych, 210, June 61(6))*

Surveys to over 10,000 soldiers were administered. Soldiers of both groups were asked if they had received care for a mental health problem in the previous month. Risk of mental problems included a PTSD Checklist, incidence of aggressive behavior, alcohol misuse and of family stressors. At both three and 12 months post deployment a higher proportion of active duty soldiers reported at least one type of mental health problem than National Guard soldiers. National Guard soldiers reported higher utilization of mental health care than active duty soldiers. The conclusion was that not only did active duty soldiers with a mental problem utilize lower rates of mental health services but also had higher feelings of self-stigma. Therefore more effort should be made to allow access to such care in active duty personnel. *("Trends in Mental Health Services Utilization and Stigma in Soldiers from 2002-2011, Quanta P. J. et al, www.ncbi. nim.hihl.gov.)*

Stigma on college campuses

Since major depression and bipolar disease are generally DIAGNOSED in the third decade of life, many people are already at a vulnerable and critical time of their lives when they are diagnosed. Virginia Werner, a college student herself, wrote an essay in PsychCentral entitled "I don't want my friends to think I'm crazy: The Stigma of Bipolar Disease on the College Campus."

Finding students willing to talk was difficult for the author. Finally she came across a student who stated the following: "My friend is dating this one crazy girl, she's so bipolar. You should try interviewing her."

The author says, "This just further proves my point. People my age don't know the first thing about mental illness."

She finally found two students at her university with prior diagnoses of bipolar disease. They expressed fear of others knowing. "I don't want my friends to think I'm crazy," said one. One was thinking of ways to commit suicide and the other said he was going to drop out of school.

As a result of Werner's intervention, one of the students is now seeing a psychiatrist monthly and a psychologist weekly and both are on medication. "It's about accepting …your life and letting go of the residual negative stimuli," said one.

Some of Werner's recommendations to the students included the work of Erica Freeman, clinical therapist and social worker who outlines four steps for people with bipolar disease: Recognition of signs of lows or highs in order to seek treatment; cognitive therapy to change thoughts into something constructive to distract from the mood; improving communication skills; and, finally, meditative or mindfulness therapies such as yoga.

Freeman says that people with the disorder can beat the stigma by realizing "it's possible to manage it effectively enough that it doesn't have to change their ability to do anything they want to do in their life."

Stigma in society

If you're admitted to the hospital for appendicitis, should the first diagnosis listed by your surgeon on the Problem List be bipolar disease? It often is, and I say this is outrageous. This has great significance for insurance billing and unquestionably violates patient confidentiality. Any caregiver with legal access to your chart will know facts about your psychiatric history that they have no business knowing. Unfortunately, the disclosure keys them in on your bipolar disease and distracts them from your main medical or surgical problem.

A monograph by the Depression and Bipolar Support Alliance (DBSA) speaks to "Fighting Stigma." A survey of 1200 American adults of all demographics revealed that 25% had misconceptions about bipolar disease. For example, they believe that people with bipolar disease are not like everyone else, should not have children, are easy to spot in the workplace and cannot live normal lives even when treated. In addition, two-thirds of the people surveyed felt that mood disorder medications are habit forming.

Furthermore, the DBSA monograph concludes that people in the workplace with bipolar disease face greater stigmatization than people with physical disabilities or limiting conditions.

Self-stigma

Self-stigma may be the worst corollary to stigma itself. Self-stigma means that a.) you are aware of the negative social beliefs, b.) you agree with them, and c.) you apply them to yourself. This leads to lowered self-esteem and inability to achieve life goals — a sort of 'why bother?' attitude, even when evidence exists that proves those negative beliefs are misguided.

In one study of 264 psychiatric patients admitted with either Bipolar I or Bipolar II showed that self-stigma had a significant impact on both the impairment of functioning and the patient's social adjustment seven months later. (*Stigma as a Barrier to Recovery: Adverse Effects of Perceived Stigma on Social Adaptation of Persons Diagnosed with Bipolar Affective Disorder," Deborah A. Peflick, Ph.D., et al, Psychiatric Services 2001*)

In another retrospective study over forty years, individuals diagnosed as having mental illness are socially stigmatized by employers, families of patients, mental health workers themselves, landlords, etc. Because persons with mental illness internalize their disease they anticipate rejection by others and develop methods of coping that includes secrecy and withdrawal from social interaction. They may limit their social interaction to family members who accept their stigma. Self-stigma was worse in those who relied solely on family members than those who could share their concerns outside the household. Withdrawal becomes a coping mechanism and delays recovery from any given episode of acute depression or mania. The most serious outcome of such self-stigma is avoidance of seeking treatment. *(ibid)*

The first step in challenging societal beliefs is to challenge them in ourselves.

Those of us with either of these diseases feel we have to be on guard. We feel we have to be careful about what and to whom we reveal information about our history and condition. Once you let the cat out, so to speak, you may feel that some acquaintances, friends or family members look at you as damaged goods. You may perceive this even if it is not true. My advice is to start by respecting yourself. Decide that holding yourself in high regard is important and valuable. You can remain 'on guard,' and careful about how you share information, but think of yourself as smart and strategic, rather than hiding and not wanting to be found out.

You do need your support team, however. The more you can step up with a determination to live your life well, and wisely, you'll know that you need to rely on others. Your significant other, spouse or closest family member needs to be involved in your care. They may be able to spot the beginning of a high or low earlier than you can recognize it. They need to know your medications, their side-effects and may even need to monitor your compliance, sometimes by doing a pill count from your prescription bottles. They also need to monitor your self-medication such as more than moderate alcohol consumption, marijuana or illicit drugs. In general, any use of these will be frowned upon by a competent psychiatrist. Occasionally your partner or main support team member may need to attend a session with your psychiatrist.

Creating and relying on your support team takes courage, determination and humility. Getting there will help you remove self-stigma about bipolar disease.

Conclusion

I think about social conscience a great deal in my daily living. To me, having a social conscience means not affecting others in a negative way. Besides the Hippocratic oath I took when I became a doctor, "First, do no harm," my interpretation of social conscience includes simple things like not saying hurtful things, not cutting off other drivers, not yelling at nurses (and when I have, apologizing), drawing attention if undercharged at a restaurant and, in larger way, following the Ten Commandments.

For people with bipolar disease, having a social conscience also means accepting the disease and deciding to live as well as you can despite it. This requires learning about your disease so that you are responsible for yourself and better able to regulate your behavior. It also means taking responsibility for your actions and allowing others to help in your care. Ultimately those with bipolar disease need to prevent adverse consequences to themselves, their loved ones and others. This is what I mean by having a strong sense of social conscience if you are living with bipolar disease.

If you have bipolar disease, here are 7 steps to take, starting today, to live your life with a social conscience.

1. Decide to be pro-active.
2. Make sure you are under the care of a competent psychiatrist.
3. Educate yourself about bipolar disease.

4. Surround yourself with a committed support team.

5. Listen to your support team and don't feel threatened by them.

6. Understand the dangers of self-stigma and work to change your beliefs.

7. Take steps to manage your career and life situations strategically.

Living with bipolar disease does not have to mean hiding in secrecy. I encourage you to follow these seven steps to help you meet the challenges of living with bipolar disease, and to live a life that is full, joyful and meaningful.

About the Author

Originally from Washington, D.C., Paul Golden, M.D., received his B.S. from Yale University, his M.D, from Washington University School of Medicine in St. Louis, his internship and residency from the University of California at San Francisco and his Fellowship in nephrology from Barnes Hospital of Washington University School of Medicine. He became one of the first practicing nephrologists in Modesto, California, where he lives with his wife, Sue, and their two toy poodles.

Dr. Golden retired from his medical practice in 2013 to focus on sharing his message about living successfully with bipolar disease.

Paul Golden, MD, *The Bipolar Physician,* is available for speaking engagements.

His memoir, ***The Bipolar Physician: A Story of Struggle, Survival and Success*** will be released in 2016.

Visit Dr. Golden's website at: www.mdgolden.com or connect with him at paul@mdgolden.com

Made in the USA
San Bernardino, CA
28 April 2017